My Challenge

From the Depths to the Heights

Barb Derrick

"Barb Derrick, who has walked through the
valley of depression and been thrust to
the perilous peaks of mania, shares her
sensitivities and insights with her poetry."

- From the foreword of James H. Thomas, MD

authorHOUSE®

AuthorHouse™
1663 Liberty Drive
Bloomington, IN 47403
www.authorhouse.com
Phone: 1-800-839-8640

First published by AuthorHouse 5/10/2011
ISBN: 978-1-4567-5967-4 (sc)
ISBN: 978-1-4567-5968-1 (e)

Printed in the United States of America

*Any people depicted in stock imagery provided by Thinkstock are models,
and such images are being used for illustrative purposes only.
Certain stock imagery © Thinkstock.*

This book is printed on acid-free paper.

*Because of the dynamic nature of the Internet, any web addresses or
links contained in this book may have changed since publication and
may no longer be valid. The views expressed in this work are solely those
of the author and do not necessarily reflect the views of the publisher,
and the publisher hereby disclaims any responsibility for them.*

Cover design by Amy Sagola Bennett and Angela Simonson

Dedicated
to
Helen Nyquist Weekes
and my daughter, Cindy A. Wengert

FOREWORD

People, who have gone places seen things, experienced events, had feelings and imaginings that the rest of us have not had, can broaden, deepen and enlighten our awareness of our own experiences when they share with us.

Barb Derrick, who has walked through the valley of depression and been thrust to the perilous peaks of mania, shares her sensitivities and insights with her poetry. Over the years that we have worked together Barb has frequently brought poetry, both literally and figuratively, to our meetings. The poetry collected in this book is a sampling that helps all of us live more richly.

By expressing powerful feelings in a controlled manner, we can gain some understanding of them along with safety from extreme, dangerous and uncontrolled actions or feelings. Enjoy the collection of poetry in this book as they excite, provoke, and nurture you.

James H. Thomas, MD

ACKNOWLEDGEMENTS

I would like to thank my friend and fellow poet, Alice I. Irvin who edited these poems and encouraged me in my quest for publication.

I am thankful for my doctor's listening, commenting, and encouraging words on my poetic works for many years. James M. Thomas, MD, Professor and Author.

I want to thank my teacher and friend, Murray Bodo, who is a priest, poet, professor, author of essays, meditations and his twentieth book, "The Earth Moves At Midnight". He has given me positive advice and encouragement throughout the many years.

My thanks goes to my poetry group, Creative Hearts, for their constant aid and understanding, editing and loving comments.

My special thank you to my two nieces for their creative interpretation of the cover material.

My thanks also to my family members who always supported my writing especially as this book progressed.

CONTENTS

LIDO BEACH

The beach is special – a sheltering cove
only sea gulls to see what is seen
abreast of the water – abreast of the sea
everyone here lives two breasts from the sun.

11/22/83

TURBULENCE

Blue waters shining – warm with the sun
shielding the turbulent sea life below
how sweet is her smile – how warm and serene
shielding the turbulent she life below.

12/12/83

FUTURE INVESTMENT

In the factories
of America
amidst the noisy busyness
of assembly,
we mold the precious metal
vital to the growth of the nation,
for HIGH wages;
In the day care centers
of America
amidst the noisy busyness
of early childhood learning,
we mold the precious child
vital to the growth of the nation,
for LOW wages.

One product is ready – in the now
One product is ready – in the future
What is our country's message?
don't invest in the child –
there's no future!

2/16/85

BEHOJA

When mind dwells in lawn
Lost in blades of confusion
Mother Earth observes
And calmness reveals path.
We're flower parents
All petals blown away
Listen, observe sky
Let children discover why.
Small bird sings a song
Calls to sad one at the dawn
For her will is weak
The darkness calling is strong.

7/14/85

NOT IN SIGHT

A scattered pattern
of shiny blue puzzle pieces
outside her cabin's screened porch
a picture flutters through
the leafy green branches
from lake side beach
to heavenly ceiling
no division between
only a movement so slight
indicating a realness
not in sight.

7/23/85

NOT SICK

Once placed on a mental floor
no matter how modern the facility
you are now perceived as strange
you may as well go out in public
dressed in your pajamas
for the chemical imbalance
that affects your drastic mood swings
is understood like Einstein's theory.

You're different now
a giraffe penned with the hippos
their vision short-sighted
their trust limited
their well-meaning advice
causes a need to vomit
ridding yourself of the feelings
of resentment and aloneness.

Cancer or a hysterectomy
would bring true concern
even flowers, cards or letters
with an encouraging word
but, let's face it, dears
you're out of gear, out of sync
you're just unstable -
not sick!

9/21/85

SUNLIGHT ON THE CREEK

Sunlight on the creek
a mystique
as shadows from
the sharpened naked Blackthorn trees,
the crouching nested wild-rose bushes,
the umbrella-like baby maples,
and sticks of drying milk-weed pods
each paint images
in the stillness of the water;

she sits and looks intently
in this favorite mirrored place
to find her self identity
and the winding creek looks back
feeling the love vibrating
longing to satisfy her;

soon she sees a reflecting scene
of a young girl sitting beside
another creek, long ago,
meditating, contemplating,
lost in the quiet questioning
of life,
even then.

10/2/85

TWO FRIENDS

Two manic-depressives
meet with compassion
clasp hands for a moment
    one going UP
        the other going DOWN
tomorrow it may be
    the other way around.

10/13/85

UNDERSTANDING IT

You have everything
and after a fantastic high
of buying, selling and investing
you're suddenly in the depths
of depression and guilt
you've almost depleted your inheritance
in a manic elevated mood
now you're down at the bottom
of your chemical imbalance
you've retreated from the world
suffering the self-hate hell
your friends think you're just ill
but I know where you are
I understand the madness felt
accomplishing the top
you now hate yourself
not able to make a decision
 you've become an empty shell.

You're controlling your illness now
after two stays in the mental ward
but only because you pushed
to understand the reason
for twenty years of elation-depression
and of trying to relieve your mate
 from the strain of
dealing with such re-occurring tensions.
You have the choice
of "toughing it out" at home
but what have you learned

in controlling such mood-swings again?
now, when you feel yourself retreating
becoming very down
you call your doctor
as soon as you can admit it
work on medication
re-learning about self-hate again.
You're feeling well today
the best you've felt in a very long time
but you know the chemical-imbalance
is still there to cope with
and maybe tomorrow will trigger
your mood to zoom downward
but you've found help and , at last,
you understand it.

10/13/85

AN OLD-PEOPLE

I don't want to be an old-people
they're everywhere you look down here

       on the beach
       at the grocery
       on the sidewalks
       at restaurants
       at shopping centers

coming and going
taking their time
all hurried-out
only
now he has the gout and
she fusses with his food
and with him;

I've definitely decided I'll never be an old-people

       every time I laugh at one of their jokes
       or listen to an amusing story
       or confide as they sleepily listen
       or answer another friendly greeting
       or wonder at the grouchy guy on the bench,

I realize there are no old-people here
as I advance to take my place.

                    12/7/85

AT REST

Partaking of my sustenance
while lazing on a balcony
overlooking acres and acres
of blue-green water
of paint-whitened sea foam
of graying sea gulls
all at rest
yet
moving constantly,

I wondered if I would remember thus
partaking of my sustenance
overlooking acres and acres
of orchard land
of manufacturing area
of workman – of my man,
at rest yet on constant move,
at rest yet on constant move.

12/7/85

THE AGE OF GRAY

Antique family rings

on cultured lady's old fingers

diamonds and rubies

molded and mounted in keep-sake form

now fit a bit looser

as the flesh ebbs away

and the dullness

of rings

matches

the age of gray

12/7/85

A TRADE

Searching for shells
by the sea
can take hours
of walking
stopping
staring
and finally
spotting a hand full
of the particular shape
that satisfies
the eye;
in the meantime,
the surf resurfaces
the sky shines a sharp blue
down to the horizon,
the pelicans fly and eat
sit and watch;

and the hours go by…
pleasantly
peacefully
and the rest of the
world disappears in
my mind
allowing a slowing down
time
inside and outside
of my body,

as I trade finding
shells
for finding
a tombstone.

12/8/85

TRAVELERS

An oasis exists – where
we travelers of many races and religions
struggle through the sinking grains of quartz
the more agitated we become
the less we gain
and the day creeps on
until the sunset comes
our labor is over
we've reached
the holy water –
the sustenance for living –
but
life is gone.

12/8/85

SO EASY

Are you here beside me
walking the tide in
on the beach
as free as a seagull
your spirit penetrates one medium
to another
shining starfish to
gliding pelican,
while I travel the earth
you follow on your level.

Your freedom tempts
relinquishing control
letting darkness take the toll
the only difference
would be the disappearance
of a microscopic blip
on a radar screen
somewhere.

It would be so easy
to rid me of the frustrations
of another problem every day
that I'm not supposed to
think about,
only take care of me, they say,
where's the challenge, the zest
I knew?

I may allow your illness
to enter and take me
out your door.
To fly in the eternally blue sky
play golf on the emerald greens
sail on the warm blue Gulf waters,
so easy
so easy....

12/9/85

THE SAME HAND

Cremating living Jews in the morning

Feeding wild birds in the afternoon

all in the same day
in the life of a man
dedicated to a cause of
another man's nightmare.

The first was an order
done with no thought
the second action
the only thought allowed.

The hand that pulled the switch
reconciled his inhumanity
by using the same hand
to feed the
wild birds.

12/18/85

TREASURE

A fresh young flower
    mated
with an adventurous Lochinvar
who rushed off in search
    of treasure,
time and time again
he rode off
only to lose
his King's treasure
then gallop home
    more slowly
to his maiden;
she sat patiently in her window
hands sore with the scrubbing
of others' pots and pans,
she treasured him
    oh, so truly,
when each journey repeated
they asked the King's Treasurer
    for help
he paid all of the losses
in return
    for their service
    forever,
family and friends cried
    when they saw
these two branded, so young,
disgraced in the eyes
of the kingdom.

2/2/86

FIRST

It's fun to have a granddog
they seldom cry
or burp or clutter up the house
with toys or Pampers mess,
they come when called
and lick your hand
worship at your feet
and don't talk back
or get a tummy ache,
you bathe them very seldom
and spray for ticks or fleas
they love whomever feeds them
and follow in your steps,
but if ever we were lucky
and had a grandchild, too,
I'd remember that our granddog
was first, before the new!

4/14/86

DAWNING FEAR

Is she breaking down again
after weeks of normalcy?
she's so uptight
her pen won't stop on the page
writing on with an urgency,
the unconscious thoughts
coming through
to challenge her
tire her
with a compulsiveness unfelt
for more than a year,
frightened, she attempts to stop
then creeps back again
to the one lighted room
with pen in hand,
and the quietness
of this writing night
avoids her tomorrow
with a dawning fear.

4/15/86

RELEASE

A collection of toys
begun only last year
are satisfying
to her soul,

her friends are:
a heavy metal red caboose
a kawala bear named Violet
a white soft cuddly bear
a child's book of poems
and
a small artificial tree
with multi-colored bows
and tiny lights,

these special toys
are instrumental
in the release of
the bad child inside
she's carried around for years
she may learn
she's good.

4/15/86

READY EXPERTS

The heirloom rock-a-bye bed
graces our living room
filled with growing greenery,
once filled with our babies
spaced one at a time,
my sister and I shared our antique
for six newborn infants
2 male and 4 female,
but this generation
hesitates
waits
to make the decision,
don't they know now?
we're how-to-raise-children experts
we've made the mistakes
now we will impart
this knowledge to them willingly
if they would only stop thinking
and produce!

4/15/86

THE TEA LEAVES

When the man of the house
had the creek bulldozed
and straightened
several years ago
the woman of the house
silently endured
the ravaging
of "her" creek,

she runs to her favorite spot
each Spring and searches,
for the peppermint tea leaves
to return by the creek,
only to find --
something lost.

4/24/86

ONLY THE SCAR

Only the scar was there

when she dressed in the morning light

when she undressed at night, for

part of her Self was gone

her womanhood

so warm

to the touch

his touch

was gone

his eyes averted

reinforcing her opinion

of her worth

till only the scar was there

between them.

5/1/86

BEHOJA – TONKA

Her lovely straw hat

Purchased on Hawaiian trip

Worn to family wedding,

Prompted Reunion cousins

Hats on every head,

Being different has pain.

5/2/86
(Japanese Poetry)

UNENDING

Swirling, a whirling dervish, of words
filling, over-spilling, her mind
an unending tornado of
syllables and rhyme
unrelenting in the dark night
driving her up from her bed
to release the agony of fire
till finally on paper,
poetry compulsion
turned off
at last

5/15/86

THE BREATH OF LIFE

A sea of black robes
hats cocked
tassels in motion
each head high – proud
each heart beating – fast
minds and horizons
stretched to bursting
new knowledge, new outlook
expanded Self
some ready at the precipice
to fly
some drawing back a bit
accumulating
the self-worth needed
to step in air
unsupported
and feel the breath
of life
buoying them up to the heights
where the Chariots of Fire
await.

5/19/86

THE GIFT OF WONDER

He appeared
and all wondered
at the simpleness of his garb
a Franciscan priest
in his robe of rough texture
hood resting, head bare
    with sandal-shod feet:

    He neared
his short trimmed graying beard
    tanned Italian complexion
soft brown sparkling eyes
framed the smile of St. Francis;

He spoke
and all listened
to this creator, teacher
diviner of words;

He gave
his gift of words
    and wonder appeared in their eyes
and wonder is the beginning.

5/19/86

A TINY SHADOW

He holds tightly to your hand
when you visit at the Home
a tiny shadow on the bed
speaking words that disconnect
but occasionally reflect
the brilliant mind
that once was there;

this frightened little lamb
once so courtly in manner
and respected on campus
now rarely smiles;

when time to depart
a kiss on his forehead
brings memories back
then a weak smile appears
signaling goodbye
confirming this visitor's return.

5/24/86

S-O-O TIRED

The days go by
like the tick of a clock
till one tock unlocks
a snarling tigress,
those around her
cower in surprise
and dismay
as she bites and scratches
tears their souls
until the blood drips
and tears flow;

returning from an emotional high
chemical dust and pollen dust
have re-set her switch
and
the brain slipped back into animalistic time;

She's s-o-o- GODDAMNED tired of it!

5/24/86

PAY AT THE DOOR

Best friends are rare
but lately
I seem to be collecting
quite a number of them
so I'll mention just a few:
    one reaches me
    on a head to head basis,
    one reads me
    with X-ray vision,
    another knows and hears
    every sniffle and sigh,
    one deals with me
    woman to woman,
    one male communes with me
    as a whole person;
my devoted friends, in my middle-age,
seem to carry MD and PHD labels
and
I need to pay them
at the door.

5/31/86

GAMES

Competitive spirits
clothed in service blue
projected into the heavens
from a water-bound deck
mastering a swift machine
created to destroy
a similar swift machine
the winner – the Top Gun;

the thrill to these young warriors
is in the chase
the jet-paced race
to out-maneuver
today's enemy in the skies
until the whirling twisting
foreign piece of metal
is frozen for a split second
in the other's Right sights;

And the game becomes real
an immediate choice –
a warning or a thumb press,
which prevails
in this dog fight above the clouds?
"Kill or be killed" training
drilled in the cerebellum
of young men born in innocence.

6/8/86

RELEASE AND REPLACE

"And the glory of the Lord
shown round about me,"
as I stand transfixed
on my back porch
amidst the beauty and violence
of alternate bright flashes, black thunder
in the rumbling night skies surrounding me;

as the steady rain falls
each sky-opening lightning bolt
attracts me
even as it frightens me;

but the Glory entices,
a need begins to arise in me
to relinquish my close companion,
my shield these past few years,
my own raging storm
and release it
with soft raindrops
and replace it
with warm sunshine.

6/11/86

A LITTLE LUMP

"Just a little health problem,"
 she told me on the phone
and I held my breath – again,
 another friend had said the same
about a little lump
 just a bump in the breast
and she was gone
 within a year;

now to hear this friend
        my partner poet laureate
tell the story of a lump
        brought our writing to a stop
as life became more than adjectives
        and cheerful banter was exchanged
but the depth of friendship had grown
        and my lump was in my throat;

so my husband and I waved goodbye
        as she flew to her doctor-son
his love and protection surfaced strongly
        at the mention of one little lump
"She must have the best care,"
        also, he needed her there
her first-born was granted his wish
        wife and baby granddaughter beckoned;
this lady can only be described as special
        an honest, caring person
quietly struggling with losing her mate
        whose intelligence disease had eaten away

but her ready laugh and healthy outlook
        have endeared her to a wide circle of
friends
so the hugs she received when leaving
will be doubled, for she's returning – benign!

6/26/86

YESTERDAY

Why do we so often
in dreams deep in
the night, peel away
the years so quickly
to a time or place
where familiar people
dwell?

we feel the passion,
depth of sorrow, pain or
comfort relived again
so real we honestly touch
and find ourselves
in the hidden yesterday.

6/27/86

UNDERSTANDING –
BUT CRYING

Such a beautiful event
    bride and groom glowing
    witnessed by loved ones
    wishing their blessing
    for a union unbroken
    vows given, a promise
    "till death do us part";

Such a beautiful pair
    a young couple residing
    together as one
    asking their families
    to understand and approve
    of living only for today
    mistrusting the vows;

Such a beautiful outlook
    new generation souls
    plastic and permanent
    confused with
    solid and temporary
    parents of offspring
    understanding – but crying.

7/22/86

NUDITY IN THE NIGHT

As an infant in the 30's
    well diapered in her
    white antiseptic gauze,

as a child and entering
    the teens, snuggies
    were the eternal guise,

as a bride and till reaching
    fifty, white cotton
    briefs guarded from infection,

day and night she protected
    a girls' most intimate section
    "it" was nude only briefly,

but recent changes in self-image
    the questioned mores of mother
    have brought her the freedom
    of nudity in the night!

7/26/86

USE ME NO MORE

She's happy up there somewhere
after leaving the labor of it all
from a teen-age wedding
      to six births in a row
a factory-working husband
      escaping into his reading
      post-poning needed house repair,

toddlers, diapers, illness
      and near poverty
turned gradually into
      marriages, divorces, children,
      grandchildren returning again,

till heart repair and depression
enough husband criticism
brought anger, finding herself -
a G.E.D. first, amazing the family
then college and soon
an Associate's degree,

even then he found fault
so threatened he couldn't admit
she had a brain, too,

but the one crutch she couldn't let go of
finally took its last "puff"
as the takers watched
      she finally released her body
      like innumerable tired
      mothers today
            cried, "Use me no more!"

7/28/86

SO SHE LEFT

A lighted sword sliced through
    the black skies
with angry explosions of noise
    rejecting her death
too young at sixty, too much life to live,
    "God only calls when we're old;"

she was my friend
    I'm angry now
for myself
    for her self,
was she ready to go?
    had she planned it so?

as pack after pack she puffed
    finding confidence in campus-classes
but realizing nothing would change
    in a world where men feel threatened,
she grew tired of waiting
    for her mate's respect,

and so she left.

7/29/86

BAKE AWAY

Sitting quietly
    clothed in barely a suit
        tuning out the
            clamor - of splashing bodies
            screaming - of look-at-me children
            blowing - of shrill whistles
surrounding me,

I bake away the sorrow
    the depression
        the hopelessness
from my soul,

with application of sun,
    water
      and lotion.

8/5/86

FINAL TRUTH?

At the church funeral today
    only the positive
        and solid
            attributes
were truthfully paraded,
what happened to hidden sins years ago
    the attraction to young nieces
    and shocked sisters-in-law?
the outside person was devoted
    to his gentle memory-loss wife
        he attended
            to her needs
               to the end,
the inside person was motivated
    by sexual mores unspoken
    outside the close family circle,
did he repent of earlier misdeeds
    by constant caring
        for his ill wife
           who had always turned
              a blind side?
how false life really appears
    such pretense is everywhere,
      is one to continue pretending
        or truthfully end it all?

8/5/86

THE BURDEN

Do the creative juices that flow
sentence sensitive human beings
to ultimate despair?

The internal flame of caring too much
saps our energy
through the years
leaving us
weakened vessels
filled with tears,
only a candle shadow
shining where the
bright star shone before,
the devastation
of loss
is melting us
and the hot wax drips and splatters
on our loved ones.

8/14/86

HOPEFUL HARVEST

Who was I? Who am I now?
a child once; an adult now?
a follow-the-leader wife; self-motivated now?
a mother of three; friend now?
perfect Christian; questioning agnostic now?
committed volunteer; committed manic now?
serving only others; serving self now?
swallower of anger; belcher of feelings now?
committed to partner; communicating now?
resigned to depression; nurturing self through?
a lifetime of changes
only recently growing
a healthy garden of self-esteem
hoeing and weeding the "Who I was"
to harvest the "Who I am now."

8/16/86

LESS THAN PERFECT

A woman at mid-life,
her limbs are not broken
both lungs are breathing
no birthmark mars her face
ears hear clearly
eyes are only a bit near-sighted
she functions without a uterus
her nursing breasts are still plump
every bone joint is free of pain
but
she has a handicap
and her fierce anger with herself
for having it
is just beginning to subside,

A part of her whole person,
can she learn to like herself
despite it,
this lesion attached
for almost half her lifetime?
and her fierce anger with herself
for possessing it
is just beginning to subside,

when again it causes her mind
to slide, and the blackness
creeps in, taking over body and spirit,
can her response be to accept, bandage,
and struggle to love herself,
less than perfect?

and her fierce anger with herself
for possessing it
is just beginning to subside.

8/16/86

SOUL MATES

Oh, I feel your pain, my friend,
I tell you that I care
but you must find your own answers
and I must allow your life journey to be
alone:

My letting go
enables you to grow as an individual
and myself to manage my own person
so that we will function separately
but exist as soul mates always.

8/19/86

NO SIGN COULD SHE MAKE

The prominent eyes
in the shrunken face
were filled with tears
slowly sliding down each side of her face,

My purpose in her room was to bring her
mail,
an urging compelling me,

Habitless, robed in uniform hospital gown,
she hesitatingly asked me to use a tissue
to stop the dripping of her nostrils,
pieces of adhesive tape clung
to her forehead and met
at the middle of her nose
waiting for the feeding tube
to be attached,

I held her hand with my own insecure faith
as she spoke in confused words of her faith
and all the while
I felt her spirit begging for God's mercy
and strength
as the bindings tightly held her hands,
no sign could she make
except in her heart, and the
gentle squeezing of our hands.

8/20/86

NO MORE PRETENSE

You're fooling yourself,
   you're feeling up today
      you chat with friends
your privileges include –
   a walk on the grounds
      dinner in the 5th floor cafeteria
         visiting the 1st floor gift shop
but it's not a hotel
or a sorority or frat house
or a college campus dorm;

at 9, 1, 5, and 9 the meds cart
   is rolled out in the hall
water pitchers, paper cups and
   strictly-watched doses are given
as well as blood pressure
   and wrist pulses checked;

this is no Country Club
you're fooling yourself
just because you've made some friends
   found mannerisms in common
      exercised, classed, cried and
         crafted together
doesn't mean that sometimes the floor door
   must not be locked
      during the day
         or a cute new roommate
   may not appear in your clothes
         your shoes and rearrange your room

neighboring rooms one by one, as eyes glazed,
    she searches for her children's toys;
you find your special nurse immediately
    convey your compassion but uneasiness
      watch the staff act with caring efficiency;
after taking a long, hot shower
    calmness returns
      but reality has hit
        no more pretense
          you're on a psychiatric floor.

8/25/86

JOYFUL ABUNDANCE

She was on time for
   our appointment
dressed with individuality
   in attitude
   in flair
she grasped the artwork
   needed
with a feel of the advertising
   medium
her talent flowed
   on the page
denying the fact that
   this was a college student
hiding any insecurity
   behind the responsibility
of raising three young ones
   on her own,
the opportunity of doing what
   she does well
will feed them all
   with joyful abundance.

10/19/86

WAITING

She visits him every other day
At the Nursing Home near their home
He almost always recognizes her
Sometimes recalls a fact from their married
life
But mostly he just lays and coughs
Disturbing a loose deep-chested phlem
In lungs weakened with smoker's disease
His frail body swallows in food
Is helped from bed to wheelchair
As his intelligent physicist mind
Strains to ask what day it is
Forgetting the question even as he asks;

Her heart is full of love and compassion
For this undignified fate of her mate
Her physical and mental state daily
Await the inevitable
Her pain and anger countered with
counseling
With trips away, with compulsive busyness
Arrangements are made for his body
His return to Science;
She's prepared for the worst
But can she endure the everydayness
of waiting?

10/24/86

CLOSED IN COOLNESS

Two red rose buds
in a lovely etched crystal vase
not open to the bright sun,
drooped heads surveying
the polished wood grain
of their table home;

Other roses from the same
rambling bush
bloomed in the warm summertime
but these two remain buds,
have closed their eyes
to each other
early wintertime brings an end
to their joy of life;

Almost touching in nearness
yet an unbridgeable distance remains
two rosebuds born in warmness
closed in coolness.

11/15/86

GETS IN THE WAY

We've flown through the clouds
to the warmth of the Florida sun
healing our bodies
healing our marriage
as the mid-fifties
get in the way
of thirty-six year-old glue;

We visit a favorite uncle and aunt
the uncle our children's "growing-up" hero
but the words "bone cancer"
gets in the way;

We still roar at his unending jokes
are still amazed at his adventurous stories
adore his suffering wife
but we feel death
gets in the way;

We can't accept it
or deny it
so each visit is subtle pretense
as this huge hulk of a man,
shark fisherman, boxer,
retired supervisor of men,
voracious reader of books,
gets in the way;

We leave for home
our hearts bleed silent drops of blood

as we wonder if this last battle
with the dreaded white shark
will get in the way.

12/21/86

THE DRIFTS OF CHRISTMAS

A pure white accumulation
of curls and swirls
fills our Christmas yard,
the gusts of strong winds
bring giant moving drifts
changing the landscape
minute by minute;
the ever-present roar
drowns out
the Silent Night of the season
as we sit on our balcony
experiencing the fascination
of a tropical Christmas
and the ever-changing
white-tipped waves
of the ocean-snow.

12/23/86

A FRIEND OF MINE

My heart is
    melting
great drops
    of compassion
are squeezing from my eyes
    down my cheeks;

a friend of mine
    has just given me
a Peter Rabbit wrapped gift
    tied with ribbon blue
for my first grandchild
    a beloved baby boy;

my joy in him
    fills my eyes for her
with a stirring guilt
    for his robust health
her beloved first grandson
    stayed but a few hours on this earth.

3/4/87

NIGHTIME POPCORN

Popcorn is popping
  inside of my head
lying in bed unsettled
  I vainly try to keep
the lid on the top of the kettle
  but pop after pop
  continues,
nothing can stop
  thought after thought
and I succumb at last
grope for my robe and slippers
fumble for paper and pen
  in the darkness,
the muse has pushed the button
  on the electric stove
  under the pot of kernels
  demanding to be popped.

3/14/87

GLANCING OUT THE WINDOW

There's a brown squirrel

leaping quietly from tree to tree

bringing movement to the green branches

as I glance out of my cabin window;

there's a resort-tanned southern lady

leaping from color to race conversation,

moving their kind to the forest ground

as she glances out of her stained glass window.

6/11/87

AN OASIS

Is he a saint
with his God-given talent
for unending patience
   comforting compassion
      listening endurance
        long-suffering love?
No, he's human,
 mate of a Bi-Polar wife
with mood swings of
   hyper highs
      overdosing lows
       sulking silences
        sudden anger
          screaming fits
then, when asking for forgiveness –
   loving gratitude;

He has been an oasis
in her desert of defeat
for over 36 years
and he's tired, so –
they're learning together
   to combat the disease
      to help her control
       the highs and lows
        to help him control
          his frustration and anger;
Is he a saint?
No, only a long-supportive
loving mate.

7/5/87

ON THE SHELF

His disease was inherited
her disease inherited, too
when married young
neither one knew,
now at mid-life
children gone
she sees his other "wife"
a life devoted to work
achievement, perfection
he's resigned to her moods
swinging from top to bottom
each person in their particular world
touching minds occasionally
making expensive attempts
to communicate
only a house in common
    a bed in common
    memories in common
love on the shelf.

7/8/87

TENDING HER FLOWERS

Today
was a day
when her flowers need tending;

This sweet gentle wife
with pretty pansy face
put on her wide-brimmed straw hat
her soiled gardening gloves
her comfortable old slacks and shirt,
she needed to work in the dirt this day;

As the weeds were pulled away
one by one
suspicions, too,
left the fertile soil of her mind;

The bright flowers became unlocked
from the snarls of winding ivy
the dirt became smooth and loose
as her hands worked away the doubts;

Soon all was neat and tidy
her beloved flowers were free to grow
her heart breathed a sigh
her eyes could see again
yet were mercifully blind.

7/19/87

CHAIN GALS

Some pray-ers I have known
call each other on the phone
a chain of "who's got what" information
on the sick, sicker and dying,
they oooh and aaah at such sad news
faithfully pray for each victim,
if some happen to die
that's just incidental, "I tried,"
but when one recovers
God might have helped
but the chain gals take the credit.

7/26/87

NO MORE BLOCKS

She's perfect
the epitome of any
parent's first child
perfect grades
perfect Christian
perfect person
relatives admire
parents preen

she pushes the
    bigger and better task
        button
until finally the emptiness inside
    echoes the question
        "Who am I?"
and the long-delayed searching
begins, criticism gushes out at
those close, those dear, anyone near
feels the sting of the whip
used to mold her
scold her to
perfection

finding herself requires the pain
of the mirror
building the blocks up
from the very bottom again
crookedly but honestly un-perfect
so hard, like a tug-of-war unending
sometimes blocks stacking straight

again
the effort almost tumbles
her down
blocks tumbling all around
destroying her trying
easier to die
turn off her mind
set her mate free
her children and grandchildren at ease
no one to please, a
final perfect peace
NO MORE BLOCKS.

8/10/87

CHRISTMAS CONTRAST

Good food – good friends
a tree with gifts
piled high

Candles bright – poinsettias red
a manger scene
the center

Parents – children
grandchildren
gather

Love above – quarrels below
goodness reigns
on holiday hearth

Soup kitchen – fellow homeless
one gift each
second-hand

light bulbs bright – lonely figures
silent young couple
with child

Cautious caring – seasonal sharing
holiday magic
no room at the inn.

12/3/87

BURIED INSIDE

Her grief runneth over
as she grows larger
each pound
a tear unshed
imbedded
within obesity,
a perfectly normal person
outside
all colors matching in
clothing, furniture
and candy
compulsiveness
masking the black anger
ballooning the flesh to
slow suicide – you see
her only child
crashed and died
now she's
buried inside.

12/14/87

SLIGHTLY AJAR

My eyes are open
  aware of brightness and darkness
    as the endless days pass by

my nose, open to its senses
  breathes in sharpness and sweetness
    until becoming indiscriminately bland

3/2/85

HOW STRANGE!

How strange!
His feet are on the ground
yet he
sits upon a cloud
watching
as his weakened body resists no germ
mentally agonizing why
one bastard needle could pronounce
"You die!"

His perception heightens
as his sensitivity
strokes each scarlet sunrise,
overnight the greenness appears
the mating, nesting, newborn
bring fascination, appreciation;

Humanity passes by
blinded by a foreverness
while one touched by time
embraces greedily
the glorious sunset of his universe
his earth
his smallness;
sensing his sentence
struggling with finality
the fear, the guilt
the dark nighttime anger,
he resists any release of tears
trusts a few friends only

agonizes for the why
as, strangely,
his feet are on the ground
yet he
sits upon a cloud.

4/6/88

SPINS HER WEB

Do what she
    wants you to do
Be what she
    wants you to be.

She spins her web
only to feed you
to control and
use the comparison
of older progeny
with the younger,
you must out-perform
outshine your sister spider
she is finally spinning
her own silky separateness
you are still housed
in the maternal eternal web
weaving intricate lace
to please and satisfy
the queen of grasping tightly
her mouth spewing forth another
soft sticky strand.

Do what she
    wants you to do
Be what she
    wants you to be.

4/30/88

73

PROTECTIVE ARMOR

A black serpent
spotted with red
slid quietly from under
limestone rocks
striking with venom
poisoning the semen
of the brave young prince,
writhing in body
denying in mind
destroyed in spirit
the prince watched
dark eyes unbelieving
as flesh, muscle, resistance
fell away
all fruit forbidden now
in agony
he shed his
protective armor.

5/29/88

ENDING

The flaming sun recedes
trailing reddish-pink ribbons
remembrances of hours
past promising
no tomorrow,

such sweetness just begun
colors to bittersweet as
deepened scarlet silhouettes
tender moments gone by and
his power takes the light.

7/3/88

ONLY

I
am
was
will be
only
a
house
wife,
the
be
gin
ing
and
end.

7/3/88

THE SPACE

The ghostly illusive space
haunts her restless
days and nights
a mist searching
a filling of its place
a completeness
a smile
the jewel longed for
since a child
stolen away
impossible to find.

7/7/88

PROFESSIONAL AT PLAY

The young untried
wide-eyed boy of ten
watched each
smooth movement of cue
over carpeted green
heard the click
of contact
the drop
into leather
of targeted sphere,

the lad absorbed
touched the magic stick
of tapered wood
began crafting
his dream
schooling sensitive hands
with mathematical mind
each hit click
catch of the pocket
fueled his passion
proved his special touch,
from boyhood to manhood
practice perfecting,
he finally
achieved his ideal –
a professional
at play.

7/21/88

FORGIVE

The fullness of the moon
the fool I have become
forgive gravity's pull
uncovering raw emotion
confusing a relationship
an earth and moon togetherness,

black type covers
white parchment
eclipsing our lives
forever sentenced dark apart
forgive the fool I became
in the fullness of the moon.

7/27/88

I CAN SURVIVE

I can survive
keep alive each
night
clinging to my mate
closed eyes remembering you
how it would have been
if it could have been
youth equaled maturity
erased the years
touched me
tightening sagging flesh
exciting mind
releasing emotions
to laugh – cry,
each new discovery
surprising delighting
our differences
our sameness
a maternal love
outgrowing the womb
spreading like malignancy
surrounding the heart
time seemingly timeless
sewn together catgut ties
pretense gone
man and woman time
society's scalpel cuts
away such unlikely growth
only internal stitches
fuel the fantasy

I can survive --
will you dream of me?

7/27/88

A STONE

I am a stone
alive
clothed in layers of white
seen by peering crowds
applauding admiring
the sheen of topmost layer
I exist mirrored there.

I am a stone
alive
mired in clay of red
hidden to passing eye
atomizing victimizing
the silent uncounted pebbles
who exist in innocence.

I am a stone
alive
struck with hammer of blue
casting away painful splinters
grasping clasping
familiarity to my bosom
illumination of sun exists there.

7/30/88

THE GAME OF PEACE

Little ones a'playing
in the Christmas snow
challenge
little ones a'playing
in the desert sand
to a game
of tug-o-war
using ribbons of gold,
they pull and pull
laugh and shout
giving in and pulling back,
such fun a'watching
the little ones at war
a'playing at the game
of peace.

12/1990

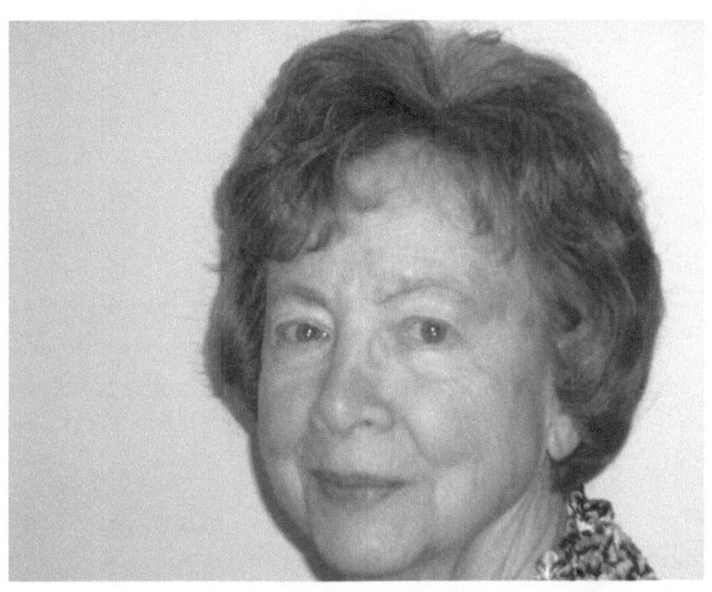

AFTERWORD

Since a teenager and throughout her life, Barbara J. Derrick (Barb Derrick) has written poetry. Dealing with the throes of Bi-Polar illness, she has put her thoughts in this book of poetry especially during the 1980's.

In 1950 she married Donald Derrick and joined him at the University of Illinois where she completed her first year of college. Together they have a son and two daughters.

During one of her high energy times in the 1960's, Barb established the first day care center in Clinton County and the 13th in the state of Ohio where she served as a volunteer chairman and member of the Board for 37 years.

She taught 3rd and 4th grade Sunday School classes for 25 years. She also had a number of firsts:

--taught the 1st year of Friends Nursery School

--organized 1st summer reading program at Putman Elementary

--organized the 1st Woman's Ecumenical Retreat for Methodists and Catholics in the County

--was the 1st woman appointed to the Clinton County Board of Appeals.

She received the honor of being named Outstanding Woman of Clinton County Ohio in the year 2008 due to her many, significant accomplishments.

Barb still lives a busy life, involved in many community activities along with her husband of 60 years.

She published her 1st book of poetry, "Christmas Moods" in 2009, and received an Honorable Mention in the Ohio Poetry Contest of 2010 with entrants from all over the world.